YOGA FOR BEGINNERS

Top 10 Beginner Yoga Poses for Weight Loss, Stress Relief, and Inner Peace

Ella Marie

© 2015 Sender Publishing

Table of Contents

INTRODUCTION

What do you think of when you hear the word yoga? Do you think of the down dog yoga? Maybe it is something you have thought of exploring but haven't made time for. Perhaps you have heard about the various health benefits for the mind and body that it offers. Hopefully, that curiosity is what has brought you here to read this book.

While some people think yoga is meditation, it is just a small form of it. Yoga is essentially a way to prepare your body and your mind for meditating. You will find that taking part in yoga poses first is the best way to prepare your body and to make sure your mind is going to focus.

The word yoga is from an ancient Indian language and it means yoking. That is in reference to a team of oxen. However, in today's society, it translates to a meaning of union. It is the process of getting the mind and body in sync. The physical practices of yoga are referred to as asana.

You will often hear yoga referred to as "your practice," and that is because it really is an individual experience. No matter where you start out, challenge yourself to grow and to see your yoga options evolve with time. Doing so will keep you interested rather than feeling bored with a given routine.

You may not think you are very flexible or have a great deal of strength right now. However, you are going to be able to improve in both areas as you stick with your daily yoga routine. The best part about yoga is that it isn't competitive. You can focus on challenging yourself rather than comparing your abilities to those of others.

If you have never tried yoga before, you may be a bit intimidated by it. However, there is nothing to be worried about. In this book, you will learn why yoga is a good daily practice to take part in. You will also get information about how to get started so you gain the most value from it.

Yoga is low impact, but it is extremely beneficial. It is a wonderful way to strengthen your core. It also helps you to get a stronger body overall that is more flexible than before. With increased strength and flexibility, there is also less of a risk of injuries to the limbs during exercise or daily routine activities.

It doesn't matter what your current level of fitness happens to be; there are yoga poses that you can take part in. Even if you have some health concerns or you are pregnant, you should be able to do some of them. Of course, it is always a good idea to talk to your doctor before you add any new form of exercise to your routine.

Yoga is considered to be low impact. This is why it is a great form of exercise for those that have had a sedentary lifestyle. It is also a great choice for those with heart problems, knee pain, or chronic back pain.

Yoga can be a source of physical and mental exercise for the entire family to take part in. Some assume that yoga is just for females, but that isn't true. More and more men are also taking an interest in it due to the overall health benefits that it offers to them. Children often find that yoga helps them to relax, and it is a wonderful way for them to get daily exercise.

Yoga can be done alone at home, or it can be done at your local gym. There may be dance studios in your community that offer it as well. It is up to you where you will take part in all of it. Look at your schedule, the times that classes are offered, and your budget to make up your mind.

CHAPTER 1
THE HEALTH BENEFITS OF YOGA

The body and mind are both very powerful elements of our overall functionality. Too often, we focus on just the body when we think about improving our well-being. Yet it is the balance of the mind and the body both working as a team that offers you the most benefit.

There are numerous health benefits of yoga – both for the body and the mind. In this chapter, we are going to explore them. Hopefully, you will be very excited to get started with yoga once you realize all that it offers. Yoga can help you to look and feel your very best. You have to put forth the effort, though, if you want those results!

PHYSICAL HEALTH BENEFITS

Let's start with the physical health benefits that yoga can provide to you. What you will generate depends on how often you do yoga and the types of poses that you take part in. Make sure you are realistic in terms of where you are starting. Don't get discouraged; give it time!

IMPROVES CORE STRENGTH

The core of the body is very important but too often overlooked. Yoga is a wonderful way to make your core stronger. It will also help you to have stronger and more defined abs. If you are interested in lifting weights, you will find that a stronger core allows you to do so.

If you are trying to run faster or to run longer, a better core can allow you to do so as well. There are very few things that you can't see a better result from in terms of physical endurance by strengthening your core muscles.

IMPROVES OVERALL STRENGTH

Yoga helps your entire body get stronger. In addition to your core, this includes your legs and your arms. That strength will also help you to burn more fat. At the same time, it can enhance your endurance abilities for other forms of exercise.

Studies show that muscles that are stronger are less likely to be injured. A torn muscle can slow you down, and it can also be very painful. The stronger a person is, the less time it takes for them to recover when there is some type of sprain or injury involving the muscles.

REDUCES INJURIES DURING EXERCISE & DAILY TASKS

Yoga is proven to help with reducing injuries that could develop during daily exercise routines or even your daily tasks. There is a combination of factors involved in this.

First is the increased strength for the core and the overall body help.

Too many people experience pain as they get older because they aren't very limber. Something as simple as reaching up for an item off of a high shelf can twist the back. Doing yard work can result in muscles that aren't used very often being sore.

We don't want to have to be overly cautious with the daily activities that we take part in. Yoga can help you to have a body that is limber and to use the muscles that normally wouldn't be used. As a result, when you do use them in a daily activity or a special event, they aren't going to be injured or sore.

INCREASES ENERGY LEVEL

Never say that you are too tired to exercise! By getting some daily exercise, you can actually increase your energy level. Then you won't feel sluggish mid-day and be reaching for caffeine drinks to perk you up.

Not getting enough exercise each day can result in you not having enough energy. A body that is in motion stays in motion. It is a cycle from which too many people can't break free. They are tired all the time because of a lack of movement, and they feel like they can't move because they are too tired. You have to take action to end that cycle.

IMPROVES FLEXIBILITY

Yoga poses will certainly improve your range of flexibility. In turn, this also helps to reduce the risk of injuries as your body won't be alarmed by the movements in certain directions.

Some areas where you will recognize additional flexibility through yoga include:

- Hips
- Shoulders
- Back
- Hamstrings

BOOSTS THE IMMUNE SYSTEM

Studies show that taking part in yoga can help to boost your immune system. This is because when the mind and body aren't in sync, a person is more likely to become ill.

TONING

Many men and woman are self-conscious about the wiggles, especially under their arms. They try to hide that area of the body with clothing. Yoga can help to tone up those muscles so that there isn't extra skin flapping around as you move or lift your arms.

LOSE FAT

Taking part in yoga can help to lose fat as it will be replaced with lean muscle tissue. In fact, yoga can be the addition to your workout that helps you shed those last stubborn pounds or get past a plateau.

REGULATED BREATHING

Focusing on your breathing is very important, and it can help you with your daily circulation. It can also help you with controlling your stress or reducing anxiety. Yoga is a great way to practice regulating your breathing daily so that it becomes second nature in your day.

Yoga requires plenty of deep breathing, and that is a change from how we normally breathe. Deeper breathing helps to cleanse the nasal passages. This can help to reduce problems with asthma and allergies.

Deeper breathing can also help with improving circulation of the blood and oxygen throughout the body. This is very important for everyone, but especially important for those with diabetes.

BETTER BALANCE

Yoga will help you to obtain better balance. This is going to help to reduce the risk of slips or falls. Most of us never prepare for them, and then they happen out of nowhere. We take our balance for granted, but it doesn't always pay off.

JOINT HEALTH

Arthritis can be very limiting as well as painful. Yoga can help to reduce the pain and inflammation. It can also reduce the chances of mobility being limited. Carpal Tunnel Syndrome can also be reduced with various forms of yoga.

MENTAL HEALTH BENEFITS

Never underestimate the mental health benefits that yoga can offer. They go hand-in-hand with your body feeling its very best too. These mental health benefits include:

REDUCED STRESS

All of us experience stress; there is no way to completely avoid it. Yet too much stress can make it hard for us to sleep, to focus, or even to be happy. It can also harm our physical health if we don't eat or if we engage in drugs/alcohol to cope.

Yoga is a way to reduce stress naturally. Yoga in the morning can help you to feel ready to tackle those tougher elements of your day that you are about to face.

IMPROVED FOCUS

Staying focused on a particular task isn't always easy. Sometimes, we are easily distracted, and other times we lack motivation. Yoga can help your mind to be focused because it is rested and it is relaxed. Mental fatigue is real, and we must take action to combat it.

ELEVATED MOOD

Daily exercise, including yoga, is a wonderful way to naturally elevate your mood. Some studies show that it can help to reduce the effects of mild to moderate depression.

Yoga increases the production of chemicals in the brain that influence mood. This is why once you get into a routine of daily yoga and then you miss a day or two, you will really miss it!

REDUCES THE IMPACT OF TRAUMA

There are studies underway that imply taking part in yoga can reduce the impact of trauma. The United States military has been encouraging those who have been deployed to take part in yoga to reduce both stress and trauma.

They believe this can help to reduce the number of enlisted members with PTSD (Post Traumatic Stress Disorder). There isn't any long-term data yet to determine just how effective it is going to be.

CHAPTER 2
FINDING THE RIGHT YOGA FOR YOUR BODY

Most people assume that there is only one type of yoga out there. However, there are quite a few different forms of it that you can consider. The key is to find the right yoga for your body. In this chapter, we will explore the most common styles for you to take into consideration.

However, before you dive into any given type of yoga, you do need to take a look at your own needs. If you have any health concerns, you certainly want to talk to your doctor before you start any yoga.

You may think that you can't take part in any given yoga due to a bad knee or back problems, yet you will be pleasantly surprised to discover that this isn't true. Yoga can be modified to fit both your fitness level and your overall physical health.

Your body weight is also something to take into consideration. If you are overweight, it may be more difficult for you to do some of the advanced yoga poses. You may find it hard to stretch to touch your toes or to hold certain poses. It can be hard to balance on one leg.

Don't let any of this discourage you, though; focus on what you CAN accomplish with yoga. Over time, you will be able to do more and more. That is the fun part of it – being able to really see yourself moving forward.

PREGNANCY

Most women find that they are able to take part in yoga during pregnancy. Doing so can help them to relax, to feel great, and to stay focused. It is important to talk to your doctor to ensure that yoga is something you can safely be a part of throughout your pregnancy.

CURRENT FITNESS LEVEL

If you were going to take up running as a form of daily exercise, you wouldn't sign up to run a marathon tomorrow! With that in mind, take your current fitness level into consideration. That is where you should start.

You can make it a goal to continue to add more difficult yoga poses over time. Don't be too hard on yourself if you need to start with the most basic poses. We all need to have a starting point. Remember, you aren't comparing yourself to anyone else when it comes to yoga.

LEARN THE BASIC POSITIONS

No matter what type of yoga you decide is right for you, it is best to start off with the basic positions. We will discuss each of them in the next chapter. These basic positions are important because so many of the poses in yoga involve them in some format.

SELECT ALIGNMENT-ORIENTED YOGA

It is in your best interest to select a style of yoga that helps your body with alignment. This will help to reduce the risk of any injuries during the exercises. If you already have an ailment, then you don't want to see it get worse.

Here are the basics of the nine most common forms of yoga to consider:

ASHTANGA VINYASA

This particular type of yoga helps with increasing strength and flexibility. It is also one that focuses on mental well-being through the sequence of movements. This style of yoga flows smoothly and involves focusing on breathing. The poses are very fast-paced.

BIKRAM

If you like the heat, this style of yoga may be perfect for you! Bikram takes place in a room that is about 105 degrees Fahrenheit. It enhances flexibility and also helps to remove toxins from the body through sweating. There are twenty-six yoga positions and they are designed for the ultimate level of overall function and health.

INTEGRAL

This is a very gentle form of yoga that works well for beginners. The holistic approach that it offers can also work well for everyday elements of your lifestyle. The traditional postures of yoga are involved and they help the body and mind be calmer.

IYENGAR

Proper alignment is the focus of this style of yoga. The postures are held longer than in the other styles. This is one of the most popular styles of yoga in the United States.

JIVAMUKTI

This style of yoga focuses on meditation and the spiritual element. It is very intense both physically and intellectually, and it stimulates the spiritual side of awareness. The foundation stems from traditional yoga teachings.

KRIPALU

This is a style of yoga that promotes the healing of the body. It also is one that works well with meditation. Mental development is also a benefit from it. Many people with high levels of anxiety or stress feel that this type of yoga completely changed their life for the better.

KUNDALINI

If you are looking for a style of yoga that increases personal awareness in all areas, Kundalini is one to explore. It can be complex, though, due to the combinations of poses that lock the body and focus on overall posture.

SIVANANDA

Perhaps a slow-paced yoga style is what you are considering. Sivananda is certainly one that fits this category. It focuses on the use of twelve postures and on good habits as well as focused thinking. It is a great option for those with health concerns, those with limited flexibility, and women in their last trimester of pregnancy.

VINIYOGA

This is a type of yoga style that puts the breathing and the poses in sync. It is a holistic approach that focuses on repetition. That is what separates it from other forms of yoga.

CHAPTER 3
LEARNING THE POSITIONS AND TECHNIQUES CORRECTLY

In order to really benefit from yoga, you have to learn the positions and techniques correctly. If you don't, they are going to be a waste of your time. They aren't going to offer your mind or your body the true benefits that they can deliver.

If you aren't doing the positions and techniques correctly, they can increase the risk of you getting hurt while performing them. Your body may not be aligned the way that it should, and that puts your spine and other body parts at risk for pain and injury.

Take the time to explore what it is all about before you dive right in! Here are some methods to help ensure you are doing the poses correctly from the start. It is easier to do so than to try to break bad habits later on.

- Practice in front of a mirror – This will help you to see how you look and if you need to change the position of any part of your body.
- Watch videos – You can get DVDs, or you can watch videos online. They will show you the

correct poses and how to get into and out of them.

- Books – There are yoga books with diagrams that also show you the right way to do each position.
- Instructors – If you take yoga at a dance studio or at the gym, you can benefit from a qualified instructor. They can help you one-on-one to ensure you are doing the poses correctly.

YOGA POSES

As you have already learned in this book, yoga is much more than just stretching. While you will certainly be taking part in a great deal of stretching for the body, that is just the start. The yoga poses also help you with balance, flexibility, and strength.

Each of the yoga poses and postures has a specific type of physical benefit to offer you. Depending on the type of yoga you take part in, they may be done in quick steps or you may need to hold each of them for a longer duration.

The approach you take depends on your choice of yoga style. There isn't a right or wrong one to select. The goal is to find something that is a good fit for your body and your mind. You may need to try a few to decide what you will stick with.

However, there are some basic yoga poses that you really do need to start out with. They will give you a firm foundation to work from. These poses are designed to give your body what it needs in terms of flexibility, strength, balance, and stretching.

Many of the yoga styles use these basic moves as a foundation for other poses and postures. They can branch out in various directions, but they mainly have a starting point with these core moves.

Therefore, it makes sense for you to learn these poses first. Take the time you need to learn how to do them correctly. It will make moving into other poses and postures that are more advanced easier for you. Here are ten poses that you should start with before you move into anything more complex.

DOWNWARD-FACING DOG

Most people have heard of the Downward-Facing Dog pose as it is the most common in yoga. This position involves planting your feet on the ground and bending your body forward, with your arms out and your buttocks upward.

It can take time to master this particular yoga pose. Make sure you don't shift yourself too far inward as that can make it difficult to keep your balance.

You want the majority of your weight to be in the legs, and that will help you to stay balanced. Strive to have the buttocks pointed upward and your heels should be touching the floor. If your hamstrings are feeling too much pressure, you can bend your knees a bit until you become more flexible.

MOUNTAIN POSE

Mountain pose initially looks easy, but it isn't! It is very important for developing your core muscles and balance. This pose also works on overall alignment for your body. Focus on drawing a straight line with your body with this pose.

This straight line should start at the crown of the head and span down to the heels of the feet. Make sure the shoulders and the pelvis are lined up too. Think of a zipper going up your back - you want to make it all tight and lined up for the Mountain pose.

WARRIOR I

Reach for the sky! That is what often comes to mind with the Warrior I yoga pose. With the arms together, you are stretching and reaching. This stretch starts out in the legs and moves all the way up the body.

The back leg is at an angle and is also stretching. The forward foot is planted and then bent at the knee to offer balance. It is very important to keep the hips facing forward with the Warrior I pose. You may find you need to get your legs into a wider stance to make this happen.

WARRIOR II

With the Warrior II yoga pose, the legs remain in the same position as Warrior I. It is only the arms that change position. Instead of being upward, they are extended outward.

Both the hips and the shoulders should be open to the side. Make sure the front thigh is parallel with the floor. This is going to generate quite a burn!

EXTENDED SIDE ANGLE

It can be difficult to complete the Extended Side Angle pose in the beginning. However, as your flexibility and your balance improve, it will become much easier.

Your back leg needs to be extended and stretched, with the heel flat. The front leg needs to be planted and the knee bent. Slowly lean to the side so that the arm on the side of the planted foot is placed flat on the floor. The other arm is straight up into the air.

When you first try this yoga pose, you may need to place your forearm on your thigh rather than placing it flat onto the floor. This is going to help you with balance. Continue to work on flexibility so that you will eventually be able to place it onto the floor. Make sure you keep the torso pointed towards the ceiling and not towards the floor.

TRIANGLE

The Triangle yoga pose is very similar. However, instead of the front leg being bent at the knee, it is extended and angled back. However, the body is bent at the waist forward. This can be a very tricky balancing act at first!

The forearm is going to be planted on the floor with the other arm extended into the air. Work as much as you can to make the arms are parallel. Think of them as a straight line – one on the floor, then your shoulders, and then the other arm.

CAT-COW STRETCH

One of the most important poses for you to master when you begin yoga is the Cat-Cow Stretch. It is a good one to take part in if you have chronic back pain. This is a type of pose that is very good for your overall spinal health.

Start out on your mat on all fours making sure your back is straight and your shoulders are facing forward. Hold your head upward and focus on taking long breathes in and out.

Slowly, put the head downward and roll the back. Focus on stretching the neck, back, and buttocks. Make sure you get up from this pose slowly.

STAFF POSE

This is similar to the Mountain pose for yoga, but you will be sitting down to perform it. Sit with your legs together but extended outward. Your arms should be by your side with the palms flat on the floor.

Focus on keeping the body properly aligned throughout this yoga pose. The back and the abs should be straight. Make sure your buttocks are flat on the floor.

COBBLER'S POSE

Many people are familiar with Cobbler's pose as it is a common stretch for any form of exercising. Sit with your feet drawn in and touching each other. Your knees will not be bent, and you want them to be as close to the ground as possible.

Try to reach your feet without bending your back or your abs. Focus on extending your arms to accomplish this task while keeping the other areas of your body in alignment.

CHILD'S POSE

Another very popular yoga position is the Child's pose. This is because it is so important to the well-being of your body. Your buttocks need to be sitting on your legs. Bend your torso forward and lower your head.

Your arms should be out in front of your body. Stretch them as far as you can manage without it being too painful. This is a good pose to get into if you feel dizzy or out of energy during your yoga workout. It can be a chance for you to regroup and move forward.

CHAPTER 4
GETTING STARTED

Be realistic when you are getting started with yoga. Too many people are disappointed with what they can do that first session. Then they never do it again. Remember, you can start where your body is now and move forward. That is the key to success with yoga!

There are several things you need to do in order to get started. You want to make sure you are as relaxed as possible. You also don't want to feel rushed. In time, you will find what works best for you in terms of yoga. However, you will need to experiment to find out.

LOCATION

Where do you plan to engage in yoga? If it will be at a local dance studio or gym, show up about ten minutes early. Get yourself a good spot and be comfortable. Introduce yourself to others around you. Yoga is a great way to meet others with a common interest.

Try to find a dance studio or a gym that offers small class sizes. You will feel more at ease and you will get more one-on-one attention from the instructor. Enroll in a class that is right for your fitness level.

You can also take part in yoga at home. You may feel more comfortable doing so on your own. Just make sure you are doing the poses and postures correctly as we discussed in a previous chapter.

You also want to make sure you have enough room for your yoga workout to take place; you may need to move some furniture around. While you are working on your balance, you don't want any items around that can pose a danger to you.

For a yoga workout at home, you can watch videos online or you can buy DVDs. As your abilities improve, you can change what you use in order to continue to challenge yourself.

CLOTHING

You want to wear loose fitting clothing for yoga. This is going to allow your body the best range of movement without limitations. However, you need to make sure you aren't at risk with the clothing you wear either.

For example, avoid workout pants that are too long for you. As you do some of the poses, your feet can get caught in the legs of them. This can cause you to trip or to fall. Avoid shirts that are too loose or too long as they can get in your way.

Shirts that are too loose can also be quite revealing with some of the yoga poses, and you don't want to be self-conscious. Women need to make sure they wear a bra with plenty of support for yoga.

While they do make yoga pants and tops, you don't have to invest in them. You can wear sweats, shorts, sports tops, etc. Many people use what they already own so that they don't incur additional expenses.

Unless you have a medical condition that prevents it, you should be doing yoga barefoot. Avoid putting lotion or other items on your feet that can cause them to slip when you are engaging in yoga. Be aware of the type of flooring too – a non-slip mat is very important.

EQUIPMENT

You don't need much equipment at all to take part in yoga. It is recommended that you have a yoga mat. They roll up quickly and you can take it with you to a class. You should also take along a clean towel and a water bottle. If you plan to do yoga at home, you can get a mat or you can use a towel/blanket.

If you buy a mat, get one that is good quality so that it will last. Ideally, look for one that is non-slip. You will find that they are offered in a variety of sizes and colors. If you will be carrying it back and forth to class, look for one that is lightweight.

Some gyms and dance studios actually have mats that you can use. They often charge a few dollars per session for them due to the cost and for cleaning them after each use.

It is a good idea to wipe down your own yoga mat after each use. This will prevent sweat, dirt, and debris from accumulating. Yoga mats are low cost, and many people have one at home and also one in the car so that they can always access it when they want to work out.

MAKE TIME

Most of us have a very busy lifestyle, and it can be too easy to push aside what we intend to do for our own well-being. However, you need to make a commitment to make time for yoga. It will help your mind and body be their very best. You can't beat an investment in YOURSELF!

Carve out time in your daily schedule for yoga. Write it down on your daily planner or your to-do list. Yoga is best if you can do it early in the morning. First, that will ensure you don't run out of time for it. Second, it helps to prepare your mind and your body for your day ahead.

COMMON MISTAKES TO AVOID

There are some common mistakes you want to avoid when it comes to getting started with yoga. These will help you to be very successful!

- Failing to make time – Don't feel guilty taking time for youself and your needs. You can't be your best for others if you aren't taking care of yourself too.
- Giving up – Don't give up because your first couple of sessions are rough. Yoga wasn't

meant to be easy, and the results are worth the effort.

- Don't compare – If you go to a yoga class, don't compare your abilities to those of others around you. Everyone has different skills and experience with yoga.
- Don't ignore your body – If your body is telling you a pose or posture is too much, don't continue it.
- Eating – Don't eat a heavy meal right before you take part in yoga. Eat a few hours before class and then have a light snack afterwards.
- Not aligning the body – You can create serious problems for your spine if your body isn't aligned properly during yoga poses.
- Negativity – Keep your thoughts positive so that you can really benefit from yoga. If your instructor or another student points out something you are doing wrong, learn from it. They aren't picking on you. Focus on what you can do, not on what you aren't able to do yet.

CHAPTER 5
YOGA AS A FORM OF MEDITATION

Yoga is a form of meditation, and it is so much more than that, but this element of it definitely needs to be explored. Training the mind to focus is important, and it carries over to all aspects of your life.

Meditation also explores the spiritual side of who you are and what you believe in. This doesn't have to be a religion. It can be very open and free-spirited. It all comes down to what it means to YOU, and that is why it is so powerful as well as unique.

WHAT IS MEDITATION?

Meditation is a form of relaxation that connects the mind and the body. Since that is parallel with the goals of yoga, it is a great match. You aren't going to be just sitting there cross legged, making o's with your thumb and finger, saying ommmm. That is just a small part of a way to meditate.

HOW DOES MEDITATION WORK?

For meditation to work, you have to be uninterrupted in your thoughts. How many times a day does your mind wonder from what you are doing to something else? You are about to find out through meditation!

When you first start out, you are going to have to redirect your mind over and over again. In time, it will become more disciplined. You need to be able to focus on one idea, object, or thought.

What you will discover is that the subconscious is very powerful! You may think you have complete control over your own mind, but that isn't always true. However, you are going to have more control over your thoughts, how you feel, and even your emotions once you implement meditation along with yoga.

GETTING STARTED

It isn't a good idea to jump right in with the meditation part of things if you are new to yoga. It is simply too much to take on at once. First, learn the basic poses of yoga so that they are easy for you to do without thinking too hard about them.

Once you get to that point, you can introduce meditation. You won't have to focus so hard on your poses and postures, so you can focus on given thoughts or focal points of your choosing.

BREATHING

Your breathing is a big part of being successful with meditation. Slowly take in each breath and then slowly exhale it. You don't want your breathing to be too slow or too fast; try to keep it natural. However, you want to take in deeper breaths than you normally do.

Too often, we aren't aware of our breathing at all; it is just a natural part of life that we take for granted. Through yoga and meditation, you can use it as a means to relax and to clear your mind.

BE PREPARED

Initially, you may find that meditation is frustrating. If you have a fast-paced lifestyle and little patience, it will be even more of a frustration. It is going to be different from what you normally do. Meditation can drain you mentally and emotionally when you first start out.

However, as you are able to stay focused for longer periods of time, you will get deeper into meditation. You will feel thoughts, experience emotions, and feel sensations of your body that you didn't notice before.

You don't have to meditate for long periods of time for it to work for you. Start out with a goal of only five minutes. Then you can continue to add small increments to it until you are at a timeframe that you are happy with.

CHAPTER 6
STAYING MOTIVATED

If you are going to gain the physical, mental, and spiritual elements of yoga, you have to stay motivated. You have to hold yourself accountable so that you are able to give it time to work for you. Don't get discouraged – get motivated! Staying motivated is important too!

PUT YOUR THOUGHTS INTO MOTION

How many times have you thought about yoga? Do you wish you had made it part of your routine long ago? Put those thoughts into motion and make it happen! TODAY is the day to get started. Stop saying someday, and make it a reality.

TWO WEEK COMMITMENT

Agree to a two week commitment for yoga. This means that you agree to take part in it for at least thirty minutes a day for the next fourteen days. If you find it isn't for you, fair enough. However, most people find that they love what it offers the mind and body, so they continue it. You aren't going to know until you try it!

REPLACE NEGATIVE THOUGHTS

Erase any negative thoughts you have, and replace them with positive ones. You will need to really focus on doing this as you start yoga. Don't get upset if you are off balance; laugh when you are. Don't focus on not being able to reach your toes; focus on the fact that you tried to make it happen.

By replacing negative thoughts with positive ones, your entire mindset improves. You will find that you have fewer negative thoughts as you start training yourself to replace them. Negative thoughts can be toxic in all areas of your life.

Use yoga as your starting point to replace negative thoughts. Then you can start to do that all day long. You will find it helps you to have a brighter outlook and to really stay motivated in all you take part in.

ELIMINATE GUILT

We briefly touched on this in an earlier chapter, but you must eliminate guilt. If you have a job, you may think you should go in early and stay late. Take time for yoga so your mind and body benefit.

If you are a parent, you may think that you should spend all of your free time with the kids. You need time for you and to take care of yourself so that you can be the best parent to them now and in the future.

Get the kids involved with yoga too as they can benefit from it. Then you can all have a great time with it together and you don't have to worry about that guilt.

TIME MANAGEMENT

Another part of staying motivated is time management. You don't want to be rushed. You also don't want to think of yoga as one more thing you HAVE to get done that day. Instead, you should view it as something you WANT to get done each day.

Balance your time so that you are able to focus on yoga. Don't spend your time doing it but thinking about the chores, the kids, or your job. Be present in mind and body and use the time to really focus on what you are trying to accomplish.

Again, yoga in the morning is a wonderful way to get the day moving on a positive note. If you wait until the evening, you may be too tired or too busy, and then yoga is removed from your plans. Yoga or any form of exercise late in the evening can also make it harder to sleep due to stimulating your mind and body.

LEARN TO SAY NO

Why do we find it so hard to say no? We want to be helpful and we want people to like us. Yet we only have so many hours in any given day to get things accomplished. Learn to say no so that you aren't constantly overextending yourself.

You don't have to give a reason why you can't help with something either. It is fine to thank them for asking you and to tell them that you don't have the time to take it on. If you can help in another way, such as a monetary donation, you can make such an offer.

LISTEN TO YOUR MIND AND BODY

The mind and the body actually crave taking part in daily exercise such as yoga. Listen to what they are telling you. Do you feel sluggish and irritable on the days you don't take part in yoga? That is very common, and it means that such a workout is really beneficial to you on a personal level.

TRY NEW YOGA POSES AND POSTURES

Like any other form of exercise routine, you are going to get bored quickly if you do the same thing day after day. This is why you need to continue to try new yoga poses and postures.

As your abilities improve, don't be afraid to try something at the next level. Doing so keeps it fresh, and that will help you to stay motivated. Don't forget those that you previously learned, though – add them into the mix for plenty of variety.

CHALLENGE YOURSELF

If you want to feel pride in the efforts you have made, challenge yourself. The only person you should strive to be better than tomorrow is yourself. Remember, do it in a way that is positive and that benefits both your mind and your body.

TRY TO NEVER SKIP MORE THAN A DAY

Getting into the routine of daily yoga is important. There will be times, though, when you have to miss a day. It can't be helped when you are sick or you have an emergency.

However, try to never skip more than one day in a row. If you do, it will be harder and harder to get back into the routine of daily yoga. If you find that you often skip due to a time issue, then you need to re-evaluate your time management.

YOGA PARTNER

You may find that a yoga partner is what you need to stay motivated. This is someone that you can take a class with or that you will work out with at home. It could be a friend or even someone that lives in your same household.

A yoga partner helps you to stay accountable and to stay on track. You will enjoy your time with him or her, and you will know that he or she is waiting for you to get there and to participate.

The downside to a yoga partner is that it can be harder to get it in at a time that works for both of you. If it is a neighbor that can come over at 6 a.m., it may work well. If it is a friend that lives across town, it may be a struggle.

You also have to make sure you aren't comparing yourself to your yoga partner. Try to find someone that is at a similar fitness level as you. Then you can both continue to progress into more complex yoga poses and postures. Yet you should both move at your own speed for maximum benefits.

REWARD SYSTEM

If you make yoga part of your daily routine, you will reward yourself with optimum health both physically and mentally. You should also have a reward system in place that allows you get something you really want for your hard work.

Your first reward should be for keeping the two-week yoga commitment. You can treat yourself to a new outfit, go see a movie you are interested in, etc. The idea is for the reward to be something that you have earned and that you will really enjoy so that it keeps you motivated.

CHAPTER 7
YOGA AS ALTERNATIVE MEDICINE

There are so many physical and mental health ailments that a person can experience. As we get older, they are more likely to develop. However, yoga can be a wonderful source of alternative medicine.

Most people agree that they would rather treat these health issues with a form of exercise than with medications. Over-the-counter and prescription medications can have harsh side effects. The cost of them can also add up, especially if the health concern means taking them daily.

It is important to understand that the use of yoga as alternative medicine isn't a replacement for medical care. You should still work closely with your healthcare professionals. However, you can let them know that you would like to see if yoga can help you to feel better.

If you are taking daily medications, you may make significant improvements, allowing them to cut down your daily dose or remove that medication from your treatment plan. Never change your dose or stop taking medications without the approval of your doctor.

PHYSICAL HEALTH

When our body doesn't feel well, it can make it hard to focus on anything we have to do. It can make it hard to work, to take care of our household, or to enjoy social activities.

Yoga helps to circulate the blood and the oxygen through the body. If you are often sedentary, then you may have some issues with circulation. This is also true if you are overweight.

Individuals with arthritis often find that daily tasks are difficult due to the inflammation in the joints. Yoga can help to reduce the pain and inflammation so that a greater range of mobility is available.

Too much tension around the neck, back, and shoulders often accounts for chronic headaches. This can range from mild headaches to migraines. Yoga can help to loosen up these muscle groups and to make them more flexible.

Yoga may be able to help reduce these types of physical health concerns:

- Arthritis
- Asthma
- Chronic back pain
- Carpel tunnel
- Chronic fatigue
- Diabetes
- Circulation
- Fibromyalgia

- Chronic headaches
- Sinus problems

MENTAL HEALTH

Our mental well-being is also very important. When a person doesn't feel well due to mood, anxiety, or other concerns, then it can be hard to have personal relationships. It can also be hard to do well at work or to take care of your family. Any form of exercise, including yoga, can help to increase the amount of chemicals in the brain that elevate mood.

Feeling too much stress and anxiety can take a toll on us. It can make it hard to sleep, and it can make it hard to focus. Perhaps you get snappy at people you work with or live with because you are edgy. You may feel like you are always in a bad mood. More of those chemicals in the brain can reduce such feelings.

Many individuals who have been in treatment for drug/alcohol abuse find that yoga can help them to stay clean. They may have triggers that cause them to long for the vice once again. Yoga can be a way to clear the mind and to help focus on more positive options.

Many people find that they sleep much better when yoga is a part of their day. They don't have to take sleeping aids that often result in their waking up groggy. They don't have to toss and turn all night and then wake up the following day when they really don't want to.

Yoga may be able to help reduce these types of mental health concerns:

- Mild to moderate depression
- Anxiety
- Panic attacks
- PTSD
- Insomnia
- Stress
- Mood

CHAPTER 8
LIVING A HEALTHY LIFESTYLE

Yoga is definitely a big part of living a healthy lifestyle for your mind and your body. Getting them in sync is important but only one piece of the puzzle. If you want to really feel your very best and reduce health risks, you need to have good overall habits.

Even though life is busy, you need to make sure you take care of what your body and your mind need. Think about them as a machine. A car can run when it has some issues, but not the way that it should. Don't take your body or your mind for granted!

DAILY EXERCISE

Engage in at least thirty minutes of daily exercise. This can be only yoga or it can be a mix of yoga with other forms of exercise. Take your fitness level into consideration and always make sure your body is healthy enough for a given type of exercise.

EATING RIGHT

Your body and your mind need vitamins and nutrients to thrive. Avoid eating foods that are processed such as fast food. Avoid foods that are high in sugar or high in salt. You don't have to eliminate all of them from your diet, but make sure you only consume such foods in moderation.

Your diet should consist of plenty of fresh fruits and fresh vegetables. Eat foods that are high in protein. Following these guidelines will reduce your cravings for sugar. It will also keep you full longer so that you aren't overeating throughout the day.

STAYING HYDRATED

Pay attention to what you drink too. Many drink products have high amounts of caffeine and sugar in them. You want to keep your intake of such ingredients to a minimum. Avoid diet drinks with sugar substitutes as they aren't good for you.

Water is the best option when it comes to quenching thirst and staying hydrated. Drink several glasses of water each day to flush toxins from your body. If you don't like the taste of plain water, add some fresh lemon or lime to it.

Green tea is also a wonderful choice for staying hydrated. It revs your metabolism and helps to flush toxins. You can consume green tea either hot or cold depending on your personal preference.

SUNSHINE

Some exposure to sunlight each day will help boost your mood. Of course, you want to be careful in direct sunlight due to harmful UV radiation. Wear long sleeves, a hat, and sunblock when you are outdoors.

When you are indoors, open up curtains or blinds to let the sunlight in. If you work nights and sleep during the day, try to spend some time in the sunlight before you go to sleep or when you wake up.

SUFFICIENT SLEEP

Most adults don't get enough sleep each night. It is very important for your mind and your body that you do so. Not getting enough sleep affects mood and makes it harder to focus. It has also been linked to weight gain and to increased risk of serious health problems.

For the best results, try to go to sleep and wake up at the same time every single day. You can't make up sleep that you missed during the week by sleeping in on the weekends.

Make sure your sleep environment is comfortable. The temperature shouldn't be too hot or too cold. You want to eliminate distracting noises. Make sure your pillow and your mattress offer you enough support.

ELIMINATE HARMFUL HABITS

If you engage in harmful habits, now is the time to eliminate them from your lifestyle. It doesn't matter how long you have been engaging in them. If you smoke, there are plenty of health risks. If you use alcohol or drugs, then you may be in danger of serious health concerns developing.

CONCLUSION

Yoga is a great option for both men and women to take part in. Even children and the elderly can benefit from the poses and postures. Yoga is good for the mind, the body, and the spiritual elements of a person.

Since yoga is low impact, it can be engaged in regardless of some health problems or limited mobility. There are plenty of benefits from yoga that keep people taking part in it daily. If you want to have more flexibility, better balance, and more strength, this is a way to make it happen.

If you would like to reduce stress, focus more, and have a better mindset and mood, then yoga can help you to achieve it. When you are starting out, make sure you know the right way to perform the various poses and postures. You want to do them in a manner that is safe and that helps you to gain the most benefits.

You don't have to spend a lot of money to invest in equipment for yoga. Most people have clothing at home they can wear for such activities. If not, you can purchase them for a low cost. A quality yoga mat is going to cost from $25 to $100 depending on the brand and style.

Yoga can be conducted at home without purchasing expensive equipment that you don't have any room for. You can also take part in yoga when you travel for work or for fun; most hotels have a gym where you can engage in it. You can even do so in your hotel room.

Since yoga is so popular, you should be able to find a gym or a dance school that offers classes. Ask if you can sit in and watch a class or get a free class before you sign up. This is a wonderful way to decide if the location is right for you or not.

Yoga continues to be one of the most popular methods of getting fit and feeling good. It is very diverse which helps to prevent a person from becoming bored with it. You can continue to challenge yourself to try more complex poses and postures as you master those at your current level.

Getting started with yoga isn't difficult, and you have so many choices regarding the style you wish to follow. Try several of them to determine which is the best fit for your needs and your health goals.

Getting motivated and staying motivated with yoga doesn't have to be a huge challenge. Make time for this daily and you will quickly notice improvements to your mind and body. That is going to encourage you to continue taking part in it.

Yoga is one of the most popular types of physical activity that helps both the mind and body. It is undertaken by people of both genders and all types of lifestyles and ethnic groups. It isn't a passing trend; it is here to set an example of healthier living for everyone.

DID YOU LIKE "YOGA FOR BEGINNERS"?

Before you go, I'd like to say "thank you so much" for purchasing my book.

I know you could have picked from dozens of books on this subject, but you took a chance with mine and I'm truly grateful for that.

So once again, a big thanks for downloading this book and reading all the way to the end, I truly appreciate it.

Now I'd like to ask for a small favor if you don't mind...

Would you be so kind as to take a minute of your time and leave a review for this book on Amazon.

This feedback will help me continue to write the kind of books that help you get results. And if you loved it then please feel free to let me know! :)

www.ingramcontent.com/pod-product-compliance
Lightning Source LLC
Chambersburg PA
CBHW071342310526
45790CB00018B/1061